200 MCQs in Clinical Pharmacokinetics

Self-assessment MCQs in Clinical Pharmacokinetics for Pharmacy Students and Healthcare Professionals

"MedPharm Excellence"

First Edition

Preface

This book contains 200 comprehensive multiple-choice questions in clinical pharmacokinetics, aiding pharmacy students and healthcare professionals in assessing their understanding of key concepts and principles in the field.

Pharmacokinetics is the branch of pharmacology concerned with studying how the body interacts with the administered drugs for the entire duration of exposure, including absorption, distribution, metabolism, and elimination (ADME).

Clinical pharmacokinetics is the science that describes the absorption, distribution, metabolism, and elimination of drugs in patients requiring drug therapy. Clinical pharmacokinetics is concerned with applying pharmacokinetic principles to the safe and effective therapeutic management of drugs in individual patients.

This book suits pharmacy students studying pharmacology for their Bachelor's degree. Also, it helps clinicians and healthcare professionals who want to refresh their clinical pharmacokinetic information during their practice.

Copyright page

While every precaution has been taken in preparing this book, the author assumes no responsibility for errors, omissions, or damages resulting from using the information contained herein.

1. The study of the time course of drug absorption, distribution, metabolism, and excretion is called:
    A. Pharmacodynamics.
    B. Drug concentration.
    C. Pharmacokinetics.
    D. Kinetic homogeneity.
    Answer: C

2. True or false: The application of pharmacokinetic principles to the safe and effective therapeutic management of drugs in an individual patient is known as clinical pharmacokinetics.
    A. True
    B. False
    Answer: A

3. The most commonly used model in clinical pharmacokinetic situations is the:
    A. One-compartment model.
    B. Two-compartment model.
    C. Three-compartment model.
    D. Multi-compartment model.
    Answer: A

4. If 3 g of a drug is added and distributed throughout a tank, the resulting concentration is 0.15 g/L; calculate the volume of the tank.
    A. 10 L
    B. 20 L
    C. 30 L
    D. 200 L
    Answer: B

5. If you administer drug X (I.V bolus) to a 75 kg patient with a dose of 18 mg/kg, calculate the immediate blood concentration C0 (microgram/ml) if the patient has a blood volume Vd = 0.09 L/kg?
A. 200 mg/L
B. 0.2 mg/ ml
C. 200 µg/ ml
D. All of the statements are correct.
E. None of the statements is correct.
Answer: D

6. Regarding "Pharmacokinetics", which of the following is/are not correct?
A. Pharmacokinetics refers to the relationship between drug concentration at the site of action and the resulting effect, including the time course and intensity of therapeutic and adverse effects.
B. ADME in pharmacokinetics refers to Administration, Differentiation, Metabolism, and Excretion.
C. Pharmacokinetics is simply what a drug does to the body.
D. All of the statements are not correct.
Answer: D

7. Ahmad is an asthmatic patient who is receiving a theophylline loading dose of 800 mg I.V over 20 minutes. Because Ahmad received theophylline during previous hospitalizations, it is known that the volume of distribution is 36 L, and the elimination rate constant equals (0.116) h-1.
Calculate the expected theophylline concentration 5 hours after the dose was given using a one-compartment model I.V bolus equation?
A. 12.4 mg/L
B. 8.4 mg/L
C. 39.7 mg/L
D. 10.4 mg/L
E. None of the statements is correct.
Answer: A

8. Regarding "Tolerance" which of the following is/are not correct?
A. "Pharmacokinetics tolerance" happens because the body becomes less sensitive to a drug after repeated or long-term exposure.
B. "Pharmacodynamic tolerance" happens due to a decrease in the amount of a drug that reaches the site or sites where it affects the body.
C. "Pharmacodynamic tolerance" is most evident with oral ingestion because other routes of drug administration bypass first-pass metabolism.
D. "Dispositional tolerance " occurs because of a decreased quantity of the substance reaching the site it affects.
E. All of the statements are not correct.
Answer: E

9. Regarding "tachyphylaxis", which of the following is/are correct?
A. Tachyphylaxis is not dose-dependent, which may indicate that giving a larger dose of the drug may not restore the maximum effect.
B. Tachyphylaxis is rate-sensitive.
C. After a relatively short period of withholding the drug, the tachyphylaxis effect is restored (i.e., tachyphylaxis resolves rapidly).
D. An example of "tachyphylaxis" in practice is tolerance to nitrates medication that is used in angina patients.
E. All of the statements are correct.
Answer: E

10. Ahmad was given an I.V loading dose of phenobarbital 500 mg over a period of about 60 minutes. One day and four days after the dose was administered, phenobarbital serum concentrations were 13.6 mg/L and 8 mg/L. Calculate the C0, and Vd respectively?
A. C0 = 16.2 mg/L and Vd= 30.86 L.
B. C0 = 16.2 mg/ml and Vd= 40.86 L.
C. C0 = 15.2 mg/L and Vd= 35.86 L.
D. C0 = 16.2 mg/ml and Vd= 30.86 ml.
E. C0 = 15.2 mg/ml and Vd= 35.86 ml.
Answer: A

11. Given the information shown in the figure below, which of the following
statements is correct?

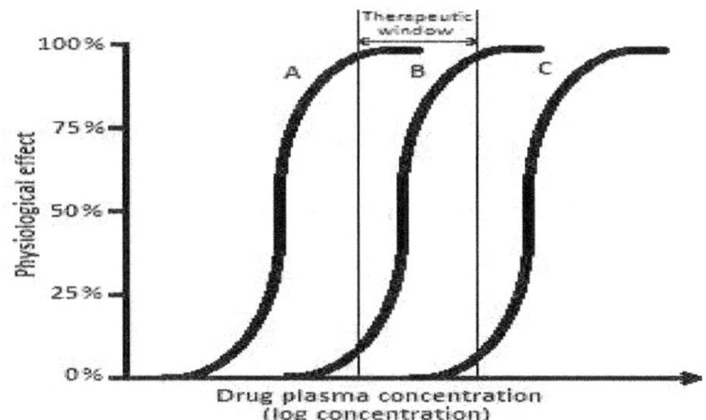

A. Drug A has the most appropriate pharmacodynamic properties of the three
drugs shown as it reaches maximal efficacy within the therapeutic window.
B. Drug B has the most appropriate pharmacodynamic properties of the three
drugs shown as a range of its plasma concentrations are within the therapeutic
window.
C. Drug C has the most appropriate pharmacodynamic properties of the three
drugs shown as non-toxic effects are achieved within the therapeutic window.
D. All three drugs have appropriate pharmacodynamic properties, achieving
maximal physiological effects and having concentrations within the
therapeutic window.
E. None of the statements is correct.
Answer: B

12. When does "Tachyphylaxis" occur?
A. When there is a decreased receptor-mediated response to a drug.
B. When there is an increased risk of side effects occurring.
C. When smaller doses cause an increased response to a drug
D. When the drug causes a faster heart rate.
E. All of the statements are correct.
Answer: A

13. True or false: High bioavailability is most common with oral dosage forms of poorly water-soluble, slowly absorbed drugs.
A. True.
B. False.
Answer: B

14. Homeostatic adaptation of unrelated systems to compensate for a drug effect is best referred to as.....................:
A. Pharmacokinetic tolerance.
B. Pharmacodynamic tolerance.
C. Physiological tolerance.
D. Behavioural tolerance
E. None of the statements is correct.
Answer: C

15. Which of the following is/are considered pharmacokinetic factors that cause variability in the plasma drug concentration and, consequently, the pharmacologic response of a drug?
A. Differences in an individual's ability to metabolize and eliminate the drug (e.g., genetics).
B. Variations in drug absorption.
C. Disease states or physiologic states (e.g., extremes of age) that alter drug absorption, distribution, or elimination.
D. Drug interactions.
E. All of the statements are correct.
Answer: E

16. Which of the following organs will mostly make up the peripheral compartment?
A. Lungs
B. Liver
C. Kidneys
D. Pancreas
Answer: D

17. What are adverse drug reactions (ADRs)? Please choose the most correct answer:

A. The synergistic effects that are seen when some drugs are administered concurrently.

B. Responses to increased drug doses required to achieve the same physiological outcome.

C. Unintended alternative physiological responses caused by the drug that causes harm to the patient.

D. Harmful chemical interactions between two drugs used to treat the same clinical symptoms.

E. All of the statements are correct.

Answer: C

18. Which of the following is/are the correct definition of "bioavailability"?

A. Bioavailability describes the proportion of the drug administered that is metabolized very quickly and thus is not available to induce a physiological effect.

B. Bioavailability describes the ability of the administered drug metabolites to cause undesirable physiological effects.

C. Bioavailability is used to describe the fraction of the dose of drug administered that is present within the body and facilitates the desired physiological effects.

D. Bioavailability is the length of time an administered drug is present in the body and thus is available to cause a physiological effect.

E. All of the statements are correct.

F. None of the statements is correct.

Answer: C

19. The value of therapeutic drug monitoring is limited in situations in which:
A. There is no well-defined therapeutic plasma concentration range.
B. The formation of pharmacologically active metabolites of a drug complicates the application of plasma drug concentration data to clinical effect unless metabolite concentrations are also considered.
C. Toxic effects may occur at unexpectedly low drug concentrations as well as at high concentrations.
D. There are no significant consequences associated with too high or too low levels.
E. All of the statements are correct.

Answer: E

20. A laboratory is conducting a study to assess the safety, efficacy, and potency of a group of drugs before allowing the agents to proceed to clinical trials. The figure below shows the dose-response curves for four different drugs from the same class of medications (Drugs A, B, C, & D). Which of the following is true regarding these medications?

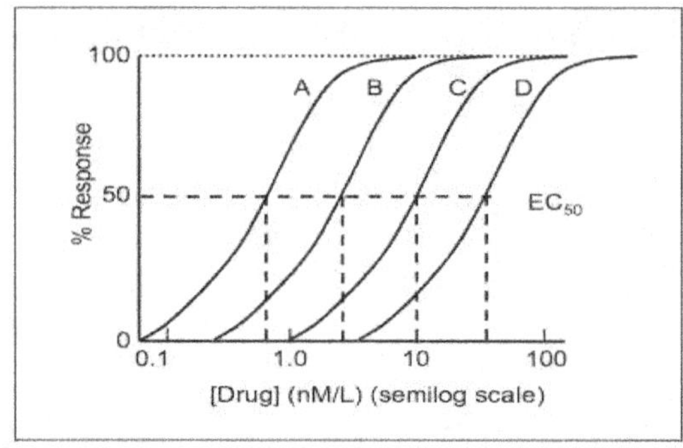

A. Drug A has greater efficacy than Drug D.
B. Drug D has greater efficacy than Drug A.
C. Drug C has greater potency than Drug B.
D. Drug D has greater potency than Drug A.
E. All four drugs (A, B, C, and D) have equal potencies.
F. None of the statements is correct.

Answer: F

21. Therapeutic monitoring using drug concentration data is generally valuable when:

A. A good correlation exists between the pharmacologic response and plasma concentration.

B. Wide inter-subject variation in plasma drug concentrations results from a given dose.

C. The drug has a narrow therapeutic index.

D. The drug's desired pharmacologic effects cannot be assessed readily by other simple means such as blood pressure measurement for anti-hypertensives.

E. All of the statements are correct.

Answer: E

22. Which of the following terms is used to describe the dose of a drug required to produce a measurable effect in 50% of the animals tested?

A. LD50

B. LD1

C. ED50

D. ED99

E. None of the statements is correct.

Answer: C

23. Which of the following best defines the therapeutic window?

A. The ratio of LD50 to ED99

B. The ratio of LD50 to ED50

C. The ratio of LD1 to LD50

D. The ratio of ED99 to ED50

E. None of the statements is correct.

Answer: E

24. The time period for which the plasma concentration of the drug remains
above minimum effective concentration is known as............................
A. Onset of time
B. Onset of action
C. Duration of drug of action
D. Therapeutic index
E. Therapeutic range
Answer: C

25. The I.V bolus dosage is 500mg, and the plasma drug concentration is 0.8
mg/ml. What should be the volume of distribution?
A. 625 mg/ml
B. 625 l
C. 625 ml
D. 0.0016 mg/ml
E. None of the statements is correct
Answer: C

26. Which of the following organs comprise the central compartment in a two-
compartment model?
A. Muscles
B. Skin
C. Adipose
D. Liver
E. None of the statements is correct
Answer: D

27. A drug solution decomposes via first-order kinetics with a rate constant, k, of
0.0077 days-1. What is the half-life of the drug in solution?
A. 0.033 day.
B. 33 days.
C. 70 days.
D. 90 days.
E. 99 days.
Answer: D

28. Regarding zero-order kinetics reactions, which one of the following is correct? Please choose the most correct answer:

A. The half-life may be represented by the expression t0.5 = 0.693/k.
B. The rate of degradation is independent of the concentration of the reactant(s).
C. A plot of the concentration remaining against time is a straight line with a gradient of 1/k.
D. The units of the rate constant (k) are time-1.
E. None of the statements is correct.

Answer: B

29. At which of the four marked points of the plasma drug concentration versus time graph, absorption rate = elimination rate?

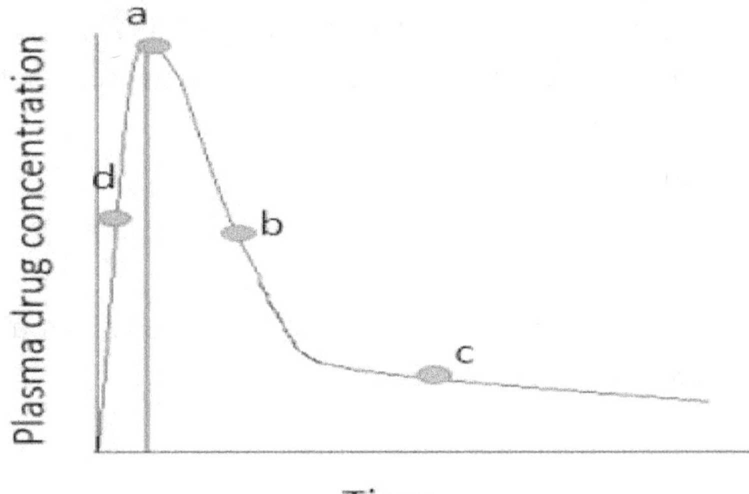

A. c
B. a
C. d
D. b

Answer: B

30. To have a plasma distribution value of 900 ml and plasma drug concentration to be 1.2 mg/ml, what should be the amount of drug that should be given to the patient?

A. 1080 ml

B. 1080 g

C. 1080 mg

D. 1g/ml

E. None of the statements is correct

Answer: C

31. Regarding second-order kinetics reactions, which one of the following is correct?

A. The units of the rate constant (k) are conc-1

B. The half-life may be represented by the expression t0.5 = [A]0/2k

C. The half-life does not depend on the initial concentration of the reactants.

D. The rate law is of the general form v = k[A]² or v = k[A][B].

E. None of the statements is correct

Answer: D

32. To achieve a target Cp of 1.7 µg/L for digoxin (Vd 500 L), the LD would be? Please choose the most correct answer:

A. 850 mg.

B. 750 mg.

C. 650 mg.

D. 550 mg.

E. None of the statements is correct

Answer: E

33. If a drug X has a CL of 2L/h, and the Cp of drug X is 10 mg/L, then
………… of the drug X is cleared per hour.
A. 5 mg.
B. 20 mg.
C. 15 mg.
D. 40 mg.
E. 100 mg.
Answer: B

34. If 200 mg of drug X is administered intravenously and the plasma
concentration is determined to be 5 mg/L just after the dose is given, Please
calculate the Vd?
A. 40 L.
B. 20 L.
C. 500 L.
D. 100 L.
E. Based on the information given on the question, the Vd cannot be calculated.
Answer: A

35. If 100 mg of a drug with a t½ of 60 minutes is taken, then which of the
following is/are correct?
A. 60 minutes after administration, 50mg remains.
B. 180 minutes after administration, 12.5mg remains.
C. 300 minutes after administration, 3.125mg remains.
D. All of the statements are correct.
E. None of the statements is correct.
Answer: D

36. Bioavailability is………………….., Please choose the most correct answer:
A. The difference between the amount of drug absorbed and the amount excreted.
B. The proportion of the drug in a formulation found in the systemic circulation (plasma).
C. The AUC relates the plasma concentration of the drug to the time after administration.
D. Always identical with different formulations of the same drug.
E. A measure of the rate of absorption of a drug.
Answer: B

37. What is the half-life of a drug in a 70kg adult patient with a volume of distribution of 700 L and clearance of 49L/hour?
A. 5 hours.
B. 8 hours.
C. 10 hours.
D. 12.5 hours.
E. 15 hours.
Answer: C

38. Tmax best indicates…………………..
A. Drug absorption rate.
B. Drug distribution rate.
C. Drug elimination rate.
D. Drug metabolism rate.
E. None of the statements is correct.
Answer: A

39. Drug showing zero-order kinetics of elimination………….,
A. Are more common than those showing first-order kinetics of elimination.
B. Show a plot of drug concentration vs. time (linear plot).
C. Decrease in concentration exponentially with time.
D. Half-life independent of the dose.
E. All of the statements are correct.
Answer: B

40. For the calculation of the Vd of the drug X, one must take into account.............................
A. Concentration of drug X in urine.
B. Therapeutic width of drug X action.
C. A daily dose of drug X.
D. Concentration of Drug X in plasma.
E. None of the statements is correct.
Answer: D

41. The half-life of the drug eliminated by first-order kinetics will be longer in a patient who has an......................,
A. Increased Vd or increased CL.
B. In increased Vd or decreased CL.
C. Decreased Vd or increased CL.
D. Decreased Vd or decreased CL.
Answer: B

42. A patient is given an I.V dose of antibiotic X (1g), assuming that the Vd of the antibiotic X is 50 L, and the t1/2 is 9 hours. Using a one-compartment model, what is the expected concentration of the antibiotic X 12 hours after the dose was given?
A. 7.9 mg/ml
B. 7.9 mg/L
C. 7.9 µg /L
D. 15.0 mg/L
E. 15.0 µg /L
Answer: B

43. A patient was given an I.V loading dose of drug X 600 mg over an hour. One day and four days after the dose was administered, drug X serum concentrations were 12.6 mg/L and 7.5 mg/L, respectively. The Vd of Drug X is?
A. 55 L
B. 47 L
C. 40 L
D. 80 L
E. 90 L
Answer: C

44. A patient was given an I.V loading dose of drug X 600 mg over an hour. One day and four days after the dose was administered drug X serum concentrations were 12.6 mg/L and 7.5 mg/L, respectively. What is the serum concentration of Drug X at time zero?
A. 10 mg/L.
B. 10 mg/ml.
C. 25 mg/L.
D. 15 mg/L.
E. 15 mg/ml.
F. 25 mg/ml.
Answer: D

45. Which of the following best defines the therapeutic index?
A. The ratio of LD50 to ED99
B. The ratio of LD50 to ED50
C. The ratio of LD1 to LD50
D. The ratio of ED99 to ED50
E. None of the statements is correct.
Answer: B

46. Which of the following terms is used to describe the dose of a drug required
to kill 50% of a group of animals?
A. LD50
B. LD1
C. ED50
D. ED99
E. None of the statements is correct.
Answer: A

47. The time needed for the curve to reach the peak is known as………..
A. Onset of time
B. Onset of action
C. Duration of drug of action
D. Therapeutic index
E. Therapeutic range
Answer: B

48. What is bioavailability?
A. The time of absorption of the drug from its dosage form
B. The rate of absorption of the unchanged drug from its dosage form
C. The time of absorption of the unchanged drug from its dosage form
D. The rate of absorption of the drug from its dosage form
Answer: B

49. Which of the following organs comprise the peripheral compartment in a two-
compartment model? Please choose the most correct answer:
A. Liver
B. Lungs
C. Kidneys
D. Muscles
E. None of the statements is correct
Answer: D

Drug X is prescribed to 27-year-old asthmatic patients (weight: 70). According to the literature, the drug X elimination half-life is 5 hours, and the apparent volume of distribution is 57.14% of the weight. The plasma level of drug X required to provide adequate airway ventilation is about 10 mg /L. The doctor prescribed drug X to be given every 6 hours. Please answer questions 50, and 51.

50. What would be the recommended dose of drug X, assuming that drug X is 100% bioavailable and that drug X is available only in 225 mg capsules? Please choose the most correct answer:
A. A dose of 225 mg drug X to be given Q 12 hrs.
B. A dose of 225 mg drug X to be given Q 8 hrs.
C. A dose of 450 mg drug X to be given Q 4 hrs.
D. A dose of 450 mg drug X to be given Q 12 hrs.
E. None of the statements is correct.
Answer: E

51. If a loading dose is decided to be given for drug X, what would be the recommended loading dose?
A. 590 mg drug X
B. 398 mg drug X
C. 797 mg drug X
D. None of the statements is correct.
Answer: A

Drug Y is prescribed to 28 years male patient (weight: 78). According to the literature, drug Y is 77% orally absorbed, 65% bound to plasma proteins, with an apparent volume of distribution is 50% of the body weight, the elimination half-life is 10.6 hours, and 58% excreted unchanged in the urine. The drug Y's minimum inhibitory concentration is 30 mg/L. Please answer questions 52, 53.

52. What would be the recommended dose to be given every 6 hours to maintain the plasma concentration above 30 mg/L?
    A. A dose of 725 mg drug Y to be given Q 6 hrs.
    B. A dose of 625 mg drug Y to be given Q 6 hrs.
    C. A dose of 525 mg drug Y to be given Q 6 hrs.
    D. A dose of 825 mg drug Y to be given Q 6 hrs.
    E. None of the statements is correct.
    Answer: A

53. If a loading dose is decided to be given for drug Y, what would be the recommended loading dose?
    A. 1935 mg drug Y
    B. 2245 mg drug Y
    C. 1625 mg drug Y
    D. 2554 mg drug Y
    E. None of the statements is correct.
    Answer: B

54. Design an I.V dosing regimen for drug B to achieve the peak concentration of
15 mg/L. Drug B is given as a once-daily dose and has an elimination rate
constant of 0.1 hr-1 and Vd of 20000ml?
A. 255 mg drug B to be given Q 24 hrs.
B. 273 mg drug B to be given Q 24 hrs.
C. 290 mg drug B to be given Q 24 hrs.
D. 223 mg drug B to be given Q 24 hrs.
E. None of the statements is correct.
Answer: B

55. If a loading dose is decided to be given for drug B (question 50), what would
be the recommended loading dose?
A. 300 mg drug B.
B. 280 mg drug B.
C. 245 mg drug B.
D. 318 mg drug B.
E. None of the statements is correct.
Answer: A

56. Design an I.V dosing regimen for drug A that has the following
characteristics: Therapeutic range 10-20 mg/L, Vd 35 L, CL 3.2 L/h. Round
the dose to the nearest 10 mg?
A. 350 mg drug A to be given Q 8 hrs.
B. 280 mg drug A to be given Q 8 hrs.
C. 276 mg drug A to be given Q 8 hrs.
D. 665 mg drug A to be given Q 8 hrs.
E. None of the statements is correct.
Answer: E

57. If a loading dose is decided to be given for drug A (question 52), what would
be the recommended loading dose?
A. 1580 mg drug A.
B. 665 mg drug A.
C. 831 mg drug A.
D. 582 mg drug A.
E. None of the statements is correct.
Answer: B

58. True or false: We adjust the dose in renal disease if less than 30% of the drug is excreted in urine and/or the decrease in renal function is more than 30%.
A. True.
B. False.
Answer: B

59. Which of the following statements regarding non-linear pharmacokinetics is/are correct?
A. The pharmacokinetic parameters of a drug will not change when multiple doses of drugs are administered.
B. The graph of the relationships between the different factors involved, such as dose, blood plasma concentrations, eliminations, etc., gives a straight line.
C. The plasma drug concentration changes either more or less than would be expected from a change in dose rate.
D. All of the statements are correct.
E. None of the statements is correct.
Answer: C

60. Which of the following statements is incorrect about phenytoin?
A. The clinical usefulness of the phenytoin half-life is limited because the time required to achieve steady-state can be much longer than the usual 3 to 5 times the apparent half-life.
B. The bioavailability of phenytoin is difficult to evaluate because of the drug's capacity–limited metabolism.
C. When the oral loading dose of phenytoin is divided into three separate doses, the possibility of nausea and vomiting decreases, and the time to peak concentration decreases too.
D. The metabolism of phenytoin is capacity–limited, so its clearance increases with increasing plasma concentrations.
E. The rate of change in phenytoin concentration in the body can be approximated by first-order kinetics at low concentrations and zero-order kinetics at high concentrations.
Answer: D

61. Which one of these is the correct Michaelis-Menton equation?
    A. $-dC/dt = V_{max} C/K_m+C$
    B. $dC/dt = V_{max} C/K_m+C$
    C. $-dC/dt = V_{max} C/K_m$
    D. $-dC/dt = K_m+C/V_{max} C$
    E. None of the statements is correct.
    Answer: A

62. In the Michaelis-Menton equation (i.e., non-linear pharmacokinetics, for example, phenytoin), when the value of $K_m = C$? Please choose the most correct answer:
    A. The rate of the process is half the maximum rate.
    B. The elimination of most drugs follows first-order kinetics.
    C. The elimination of most drugs follows zero-order kinetics.
    D. The elimination of most drugs follows second-order kinetics.
    E. All of the statements are correct.
    Answer: A

63. Non-linear pharmacokinetics is also best known as.................,
    A. Dose-dependent.
    B. Enzyme capacity limited.
    C. Saturation pharmacokinetics.
    D. All of the statements are correct.
    E. None of the statements is correct.
    Answer: C

64. Which of the following statements is/are incorrect?
    A. A creatinine clearance value of < 10 ml/min indicates severe renal failure.
    B. A creatinine clearance value of (20-50) ml/min indicates moderate renal failure.
    C. A 21-year-old female (weight = 55 kg) with a serum creatinine level of 0.8 mg/dl will have an approximate creatinine clearance of (97) ml/min.
    D. A 22-year-old male (weight = 85 kg) with a serum creatinine level of 0.8 mg/dl will have an approximate creatinine clearance of 120 ml/min.
    E. Binding of acidic drugs such as phenytoin and warfarin is decreased in uremic patients.
    Answer: D

65.   A 51 years old female patient (weight 75 kg, height 178cm) has a serum creatinine of 1.65 mg/dl, the creatinine clearance using Cockcroft – Gault equation is:

A. 43.18 ml/min.
B. 65.75 ml/min.
C. 56.18 ml/min.
D. 47.75 ml/min.

Answer: D

66.   In the below Michaelis-Menton plot, which kinetic order the graph is following in the marked place (?)?

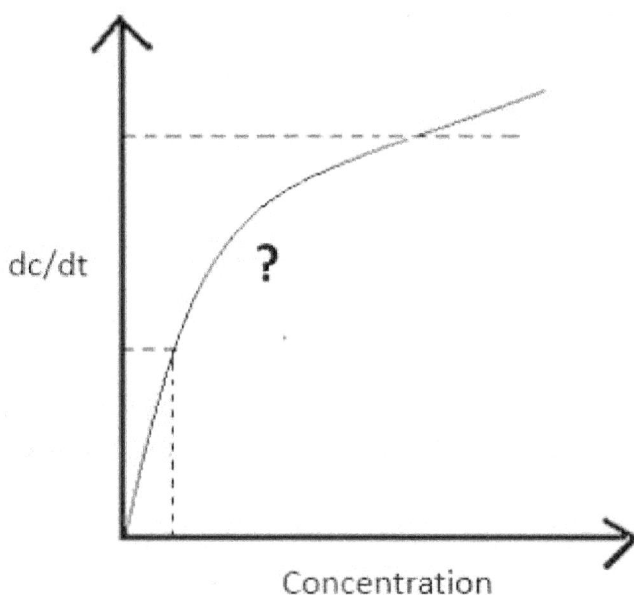

A. First-order kinetics.
B. Second-order kinetics.
C. Mixed-order kinetics.
D. First-order at higher doses.
E. All of the statements are correct.

Answer: C

67. A drug Z (which has 55% renal clearance, and a half-life of 4.6 hours) is given in a dose of 500 mg every 6 hours to an 80 kg normal patient. What dose would be used in a complete renal shutdown?

A. 225 mg every 6 hours.

B. 275 mg every 6 hours.

C. 250 mg every 6 hours.

D. 215 mg every 6 hours.

E. None of the statements is correct.

Answer: A

68. A drug H (which has 60% renal clearance, and a half-life of 4.6 hours) is given in a dose of 600 mg every 6 hours to an 80 kg normal patient. What dose would be used when CrCl 15 ml/min/1.73 m²?

A. 270 mg every 6 hours.

B. 285 mg every 6 hours.

C. 255 mg every 6 hours.

D. 295 mg every 6 hours.

E. None of the statements is correct.

Answer: B

69. The maintenance dose of aminoglycosides is 90 mg every 6 hours for a patient with normal renal function. Calculate the dose for a uremic patient with a CrCl of 20 ml/min/1.73 m²?

A. 25 mg every 6 hours.

B. 2.5 mg every 6 hours.

C. 12.5 mg every 6 hours.

D. 15 mg every 6 hours.

E. None of the statements is correct.

Answer: D

70. A 38-year-old female patient (weight 62 kg) with a serum creatinine level of 1.8 mg/dl. Would you adjust the dose of an antibiotic that is 98% excreted unchanged in urine? And why?
A. No, because less than 30% of the antibiotic is excreted unchanged in the urine.
B. No, because the decrease in renal function is less than 30%.
C. Yes, because the creatinine clearance is less than 70% of the normal value of 115 ml/min.
D. A and B are correct.
E. None of the statements is correct.
Answer: C

71. A 38-year-old female patient (weight 62 kg) with a serum creatinine level of 1.8 mg/dl. The creatinine clearance using the Cockcroft – Gault equation is:
A. 45.1 ml/min.
B. 41.5 ml/min
C. 51.4 ml/min.
D. 15.4 ml/min.
Answer: B

72. An anti-diabetic drug normally has a half-life of 4 hours and is 70% excreted in the urine. Calculate the elimination rate constant when the creatinine clearance is 40% of the normal?
A. 0.17325 h-1.
B. 0.051975 h-1.
C. 0.121275 h-1.
D. 0.100485 h-1.
E. 0.04851 h-1.
F. None of the statements is correct.
Answer: D

73. The average renal clearance of tetracycline is 3.5 L/hr, while its average total body clearance is 7 L/hr. What is the fraction of tetracycline bioavailable dose excreted unchanged in urine?
A. 0.10
B. 0.25
C. 0.50
D. 0.80
E. 0.90
Answer: C

HH is a patient who is using three drugs: drug A (Aminoglycosides), drug B (70% eliminated by the kidney), and drug C (entirely eliminated by the liver) is suffering from acute renal failure that leads to a reduction in creatinine clearance by 40%. If the elimination half-lives for the three drugs are drug A (6), drug B (9), and drug C (4). Please answer questions 74, 75.

74. Regarding patient HH, the new elimination half-lives for the three drugs, respectively, are:
A. 0.0696 h-1, 0.0554 h-1, and 0.17325 h-1.
B. 10 hrs, 12.5 hrs, and 4 hrs.
C. 8 hrs, 10.5 hrs, and 4 hrs.
D. 9 hrs, 11.5 hrs, and 4 hrs.
E. None of the statements is correct.
Answer: B

75. Regarding patient HH, calculate the new maintenance doses that will produce the same average plasma concentration produced by the original doses. Previous maintenance doses are for drug A (10 mg/day), drug B (30 mg/day), and drug C (50 mg/day).
A. Drug A (6 mg/day), drug B (9 mg/day), and drug C (50 mg/day).
B. Drug A (4 mg/day), drug B (17 mg/day), and drug C (50 mg/day).
C. Drug A (6 mg/day), drug B (21.6 mg/day), and drug C (50 mg/day).
D. Drug A (7 mg/day), drug B (13 mg/day), and drug C (50 mg/day).
E. None of the statements is correct.
Answer: C

76. Ranitidine is an H2 antagonist used in the treatment of peptic ulcer disease. After administration of the average dose of ranitidine in a patient with normal kidney function (150 mg every 12 hours), 70% of the dose is excreted unchanged in the urine. What will be the ranitidine dose required in a patient with only 30% of the normal kidney function?
A. 31.5 mg/hr.
B. 2.625 mg/hr.
C. 6.375 mg/hr.
D. 76.5 mg/hr.
E. None of the statements is correct.
Answer: D

77. A broad-spectrum antibiotic has an average dose in an adult patient with a normal kidney function of 500 mg every 12 hours. What dose will be required in a patient with only 20% if 50% of this antibiotic dose is excreted unchanged in the urine?
A. 50 mg every 12 hours.
B. 250 mg every 12 hours.
C. 300 mg every 12 hours.
D. None of the statements is correct.
Answer: C

78. Regarding Digoxin, which of the following statements is/are incorrect?
A. The kidney's primary route of digoxin elimination is via GFR and tubular secretion of the unchanged drug (75%).
B. Hepatic metabolism or biliary excretion removes About 25% of a digoxin dose.
C. Hepatic metabolism or biliary excretion removes About 75% of a digoxin dose.
D. the primary transporter involved in active tubular secretion and biliary excretion is p-glycoprotein (PGP).
E. Digoxin is given I.V or orally.
Answer: C

79. Digoxin is not usually administered I.M, Which of the following is/are
correct?
A. Erratic absorption occurs if digoxin is usually administered I.M.
B. Pain at the injection site occurs if digoxin is usually administered I.M.
C. If the digoxin must be administered I.M, digoxin should be injected deep
into the muscle followed by a massage.
D. All of the statements are correct.
Answer: D

80. 72-year-old male (weight 62 kg, and 5 ft 9 in) who has Atrial Fibrillation
(AF). His current creatinine clearance is 43 mL/min. Calculate the I.V digoxin
loading dose (LD) and maintenance dose (MD) for this patient to provide a
steady-state serum concentration of 1.5 ng/mL.
A. LD: 551 µg, MD: 211 µg.
B. LD: 651 µg, MD: 211 µg.
C. LD: 651 µg, MD: 207 µg.
D. LD: 691 µg, MD: 211 µg.
E. LD: 691 µg, MD: 207 µg.
Answer: C

81. Regarding digoxin, which of the following is/are incorrect?
A. The inotropic effects of digoxin require a higher digoxin steady-state serum
concentration of 0.8 – 1.5 ng/mL.
B. Additional inotropic effects of digoxin may be observed at digoxin steady-
state serum concentrations as high as 2 ng/mL.
C. The chronotropic effects of digoxin are generally achieved at a steady-state
serum concentration of 0.5 – 1ng/mL.
D. Increasing digoxin steady-state serum concentration to 1.2 – 1.5 ng/mL
may provide minor additional chronotropic effects.
E. All of the statements are incorrect.
Answer: E

HH patient was prescribed digoxin 200 µg/day I.V, and this dose was given for 2 weeks. A steady-state digoxin concentration was 2.4 ng/mL. Please answer questions 82, 83.

82. Calculate the revised digoxin dose for this patient to provide a steady-state concentration of 1.5 ng/mL?

A. 125 µg/day.
B. 115 µg/day.
C. 135 µg/day.
D. 155 µg/day.
E. 175 µg/day.

Answer: A

83. Calculate an oral tablet digoxin dose for HH that will provide about the same steady-state concentration found during the I.V digoxin therapy?

A. 87.5 µg.
B. 178.57 µg.
C. 78.5 µg.
D. 187.57 µg.
E. None of the statements is correct.

Answer: B

84. Regarding phenytoin and fosphenytoin, which of the following is/are incorrect?
A. Fosphenytoin is a prodrug for phenytoin that has 60 anticonvulsant activity of phenytoin.
B. Fosphenytoin can cause tissue necrosis after an I.M administration more than phenytoin.
C. Phenytoin is rapidly and completely converted to fosphenytoin.
D. After an I.V administration of fosphenytoin, there was a 90% incidence of pain or burning at the infusion site compared to 9% after phenytoin administration.
E. All of the statements are incorrect.
Answer: E

85. A male patient (weight 85 kg) was administered sodium phenytoin capsules by oral route. This patient exhibited phenytoin KM of 3.5 mg/L and phenytoin Vmax of 7.2 mg/kg/day. Compute the following:
I. The loading dose (LD) required to achieve an initial phenytoin concentration of 20 mg/L
II. The daily maintenance dose (MD) to obtain the target average steady-state concentration of 15 mg/L.
A. LD: 1201 mg sodium phenytoin; MD: 496 mg phenytoin
B. LD: 1201 mg sodium phenytoin; MD: 496 mg sodium phenytoin
C. LD: 1201 mg phenytoin; MD: 539 mg phenytoin
D. LD: 1201 mg phenytoin; MD: 496 mg sodium phenytoin
E. LD: 1201 mg phenytoin; MD: 539 mg sodium phenytoin
Answer: A

86. HH is 50 years old male (weight 75 kg, 5 ft. 10 in) with simple partial seizures who requires phenytoin treatment. HH has normal liver and kidney function. Recommend an initial phenytoin sodium capsule dosage regimen designed to achieve a steady-state phenytoin concentration equal to 12 µg/mL?

A. 428 mg every 24 hours.
B. 428 mg every 12 hours.
C. 525 mg every 24 hours.
D. 525 mg every 12 hours.
E. None of the statements is correct.

Answer: A

87. Ahmad is a 50-year-old, 75 -kg (5 ft. 10 in) male with simple partial seizures who requires therapy with oral phenytoin. Ahmad has normal liver and renal function. Ahmad was prescribed 400 mg/day of extended phenytoin sodium capsules for 1 month, and the steady-state phenytoin total concentration equals 6.2 µg/mL. Ahmad is assessed to be compliant with his dosage regimen. Suggest an initial phenytoin dosage regimen designed to achieve a steady-state phenytoin concentration within the therapeutic range.

A. 508 mg/day.
B. 2.28 mg/L.
C. 479 mg/day.
D. None of the statements is correct.

Answer: C

HH is a 32-year-old, 80kg male who is being seen in the Neurology Clinic. Prior to his last visit, HH had been taking 300mg of Phenytoin daily; however, because his seizures were poorly controlled and because his plasma concentration was only 8mg/L, his dose was increased to 350mg daily. Now, he complains of minor CNS side effects, and his reported plasma Phenytoin concentration is 20mg/L. Renal and hepatic functions are normal. Assume that both reported plasma concentrations represent a steady state and that the patient has complied with the prescribed dosing regimens. Please answer questions 88, 89.

88. Calculate HH's apparent Vmax and Km?
    A. Vmax 293. 75 mg/day, Km 1.5 mg/L.
    B. Vmax 493. 75 mg/day, Km 4.5 mg/L.
    C. Vmax 393. 75 mg/day, Km 2.5 mg/L.
    D. Vmax 593. 75 mg/day, Km 5.5 mg/L.
    E. None of the statements is correct.
    Answer: C

89. Calculate HH's new daily dose of phenytoin that will result in a steady-state level of about 15mg/L?
    A. 317.5 mg/day.
    B. 327.5 mg/day.
    C. 337.5 mg/day.
    D. 347.5 mg/day.
    E. None of the statements is correct.
    Answer: C

90. True or false: A prodrug is an inactive medicine metabolized into an active
medicine.
A. True
B. false
Answer: A

91. Ali is a 10-year-old, 40-kg male with simple partial seizures who requires
therapy with oral phenytoin. Ali has a normal liver and renal function. Suggest
an initial phenytoin dosage regimen designed to achieve a steady-
state phenytoin concentration equal to 12 µg/mL.
Note: The available phenytoin suspension is 125mg per 5ml, and the doctor
sets up the daily dose to be given every 12 hours.
A. MD is 240 mg/day, rounded to 250 mg. Phenytoin suspension of 5 ml
every 12 hours would be prescribed for Ali.
B. MD is 490 mg/day, rounded to 500 mg. Phenytoin suspension of 10 ml
every 12 hours would be prescribed for Ali.
C. MD is 370 mg/day, rounded to 375 mg. Phenytoin suspension of 7.5 ml
every 12 hours would be prescribed for Ali.
D. MD is 120 mg/day, rounded to 125 mg. Phenytoin suspension of 2.5 ml
every 12 hours would be prescribed for Ali.
Answer: A

Ahmad is a 10-year-old, 40-kg male with simple partial seizures who requires therapy with intravenous fosphenytoin. He has normal liver and renal function. Please answer questions 92, 93.

92. Suggest an initial phenytoin dosage regimen designed to achieve a steady-state phenytoin concentration equal to 12 µg/mL.
A. 131 mg/day, rounded to 125 mg/day, intravenous fosphenytoin 125 mg PE every 24 hours.
B. 261 mg/day, rounded to 250 mg/day, intravenous fosphenytoin 125 mg PE every 12 hours.
C. 361 mg/day, rounded to 375 mg/day, intravenous fosphenytoin 125 mg PE every 8 hours.
D. 461 mg/day, rounded to 500 mg/day, intravenous fosphenytoin 125 mg PE every 6 hours.
Answer: B

93. If a loading dose is to be given, then what is the best-recommended digoxin loading dose for Ahmad?
A. 265 mg/day, rounded to 250 mg/day.
B. 165 mg/day, rounded to 150 mg/day.
C. 365 mg, rounded to 350 mg/day.
D. 465 mg/day, rounded to 450 mg/day.
Answer: C

94.   In pharmacokinetics, what does the acronym ADME stand for?
      A. Absorption, Distribution, Metabolism, and Excretion
      B. Administration, Differentiation, Metabolism, and Excretion
      C. Absorption, Disintegration, Metabolism, and Efficacy
      D. Administration, Distribution, Metabolism, and Efficacy
      Answer: A

95.   True or false: Elderly people and neonates have decreased renal function, so
      dose adjustment is often required.
      A. True
      B. false
      Answer: A

96.   Which statement about the process of drug discovery is true?
      A. It only encompasses the non-clinical laboratory and animal testing.
      B. the process ascertains potential drug candidates' effectiveness and safety.
      C. It is the process by which therapeutic compounds are formulated into
      medicines.
      D. It ensures there are no side effects associated with the potential drug
      candidates.
      Answer: B

97.   What protein structures are called that are expressed within the cell
      membranes and interact with endogenous signaling molecules or some drugs
      to initiate an intracellular response?
      A. Enzymes
      B. Hormones
      C. Ligands
      D. Receptors
      Answer: D

98. What are metabolic disorders?
A. They are abnormalities in the reactions involved in metabolizing nutrients manifested in clinical symptoms.
B. They are disorders that produce insufficient amounts of energy to meet the body's needs.
C. They are disturbances in the balance of energy spent by the body on internal and external processes.
D. They are clinical symptoms that arise due to changes in individuals' basal metabolic rates due to genetic factors.
Answer: A

99. What are adverse drug reactions (ADRs)?
A. The synergistic effects that are seen when some drugs are administered concurrently.
B. Responses to increased drug doses required to achieve the same physiological outcome.
C. Unintended alternative physiological responses caused by the drug that cause harm to the patient.
D. Harmful chemical interactions between two drugs used to treat the same clinical symptoms.
Answer: C

100. Which of the following is not a means of communication in eukaryotic cells?
A. Exchange of endogenous molecules via gap junctions.
B. Exchange of nuclear material across the cell membrane.
C. Secretion of hormones into the circulatory system.
D. Secretion of neurotransmitters into synaptic clefts.
Answer: B

101. Which of the following organs is primarily responsible for drug metabolism?
A. Liver
B. Kidney
C. Heart
D. Lung
Answer: A

102. What is the term used to describe the process of converting a drug from its
active form to an inactive form?
A. Absorption
B. Distribution
C. Metabolism
D. Excretion
Answer: C

103. Which of the following routes of administration has the greatest bypasses of
the first-pass effect?
A. I.V
B. Oral
C. I.M
D. S.C
Answer: A

104. Which of the following statements about drug distribution is correct?
A. Distribution is the movement of a drug from the bloodstream to various
tissues and organs.
B. Distribution is the process of eliminating a drug from the body.
C. Distribution is primarily influenced by liver enzymes.
D. Distribution occurs only in the liver.
Answer: A

105. What is the primary site of drug excretion?
A. Liver
B. Kidney
C. Lungs
D. Skin
Answer: B

106. What is the primary route of excretion for water-soluble drugs?
A. Bile
B. Feces
C. Urine
D. Sweat
Answer: C

107. Which of the following factors does NOT affect drug absorption?
    A. PH of the gastrointestinal tract
    B. Blood flow to the absorption site
    C. Molecular weight of the drug
    D. Protein binding in the bloodstream
    Answer: D

108. Which pharmacokinetic parameter reflects the apparent volume into which a
    drug distributes in the body?
    A. Clearance (Cl)
    B. Half-life (t1/2)
    C. Volume of distribution (Vd)
    D. Elimination rate constant (Ke)
    Answer: C

109. Zero-order kinetics describes a situation where:
    A. The rate of drug elimination is directly proportional to its concentration
    B. The rate of drug elimination remains constant regardless of drug
    concentration
    C. The rate of drug absorption is faster than the rate of drug elimination
    D. The rate of drug metabolism is slower than the rate of drug excretion
    Answer: B

110. Which equation represents the relationship between clearance (Cl), volume of
    distribution (Vd), and half-life (t1/2) of a drug?
    A. $Cl = Vd \times t1/2$
    B. $Cl = Vd / t1/2$
    C. $Cl = t1/2 / Vd$
    D. $Cl = Vd + t1/2$
    Answer: A

111. Which equation calculates the elimination rate constant (ke) of a drug?
    A. $ke = 0.693 / t1/2$
    B. $ke = t1/2 / 0.693$
    C. $ke = Cl \times Vd$
    D. $ke = Vd / Cl$
    Answer: A

112. To calculate drug clearance by the area method, it is necessary first to determine whether the drug best fits a one- or two-compartment model.
   A. True
   B. False
   Answer: B

113. Which of the following equations represents the relationship between drug dose (D), clearance (Cl), and steady-state plasma concentration (Css)?
   A. Css = D / Cl
   B. Css = Cl / D
   C. Css = D × Cl
   D. Css = Cl × D
   Answer: A

114. For the body fluid compartments below, rank them from the lowest volume to the highest in a typical 70-kg person.
   A. Plasma < extracellular fluid < intracellular fluid < total body water
   B. Extracellular fluid < intracellular fluid < plasma < total body water
   C. Intracellular fluid < extracellular fluid < plasma < total body water
   D. Total body water < plasma < intracellular fluid < extracellular fluid
   Answer: A

115. A patient with renal dysfunction received a dose of vancomycin. Plasma concentrations were 22 and 15 mg/L at 24 and 48 hours after infusion, respectively. Plot these two plasma concentrations on semilog paper and determine when the concentration would reach 10 mg/L.
   A. 54 hours
   B. 72 hours
   C. 96 hours
   D. 128 hours
   Answer: B

116. Using the equation C = C0e-Kt, determine the plasma concentration of a drug
24 hours after a peak level of 10 mg/L is observed if the elimination rate
constant is 0.05 hr-1.
A. 3.01 mg/L
B. 33.2 mg/L
C. 18.1 mg/L
Answer: A

117. If the elimination rate constant is 0.2 hr-1, the percent of drug removed per
hour is:
A. 20%.
B. 1%.
C. 0.1%.
D. 10%.
Answer: A

118. If the plasma concentration is just after a gentamicin dose is 10 mg/L and the
patient's elimination rate constant is 0.15 hr-1, predict the plasma
concentration 8 hours later.
A. 6.0 mg/L
B. 3.0 mg/L
C. 1.5 mg/L
D. 1.0 mg/L
Answer: B

119. For a drug with an initial plasma concentration of 120 mg/L and a half-life of
3 hours, what would the plasma concentration be 12 hours after the initial
concentration?
A. 15 mg/L
B. 112.5
C. 7.5 mg/L
D. 60
Answer: C

120. If a drug has an elimination rate constant of 0.564 hr-1, what is the half-life?
    A. 1.23 hours
    B. 0.81 hour
    C. 1.77 hours
    Answer: A

121. Which of the following is >90% bound to plasma proteins?
    A. Atenolol
    B. Diazepam
    C. Gentamycin
    D. Lithium
    Answer: B

122. Which of the following has the largest volume of distribution?
    A. Digoxin
    B. Imipramine
    C. Lithium
    D. Chloroquine
    Answer: D

123. Which of the following is a phase one reaction?
    A. Reduction
    B. Acetylation
    C. Glucuronidation
    D. Methylation
    Answer: A

124. Clearance of which drug involves capacity-limited elimination?
    A. Theophylline
    B. Gentamycin
    C. Digoxin
    D. Phenytoin
    Answer: D

125. An example of drugs that undergo chemical antagonism is:
A. Insulin – glucagon
B. Protamine – heparin
C. Prednisone - glipizide
D. Morphine – naloxone
Answer: B

126. Regarding first-order kinetics - all of the following are true except:
A. First-order kinetics means the reaction rate is proportional to the concentration
B. First-order kinetics is more common than zero-order kinetics
C. First-order kinetics apply to exponential processes
D. First-order kinetics generally apply to high plasma concentrations (>20 mg / 100 ml) of ethanol
Answer: D

127. Bioavailability is
A. The difference between the amount of drug absorbed and the amount excreted
B. The proportion of the drug in a formulation found in the systemic circulation
C. The AUC relates the plasma concentration of the drug to the time after administration.
D. Always identical with different formulations of the same drug
Answer: B

128. Which of the following drugs has a high extraction ratio?
A. Diazepam
B. Theophylline
C. Phenytoin
D. Propranolol
Answer: D

129. The concentration of drug in plasma above which toxic effects are precipitated is:

A. Maximum safe concentration
B. Minimum Effective Concentration
C. Intensity of Action
D. Duration of Action

Answer: A

130. Which of the following is the half-life of zero order reaction?

A. $t_{1/2} = A_0/2k$
B. $t_{1/2} = 0.693/2k$
C. $t_{1/2} = A_0/2$
D. $t_{1/2} = 2k/A_0$

Answer: A

131. The k unit for zero order reaction is:

A. moles/liter/second
B. moles
C. moles/second
D. moles/liter

Answer: A

132. Which of the following is the half-life of first-order reaction?

A. $t_{1/2} = A_0/2k$
B. $t_{1/2} = 0.693/2k$
C. $t_{1/2} = 2k$
D. $t_{1/2} = 0.693/k$

Answer: D

133. Which of the following is not a pharmacokinetic parameter that describes the plasma level time curve?

A. Tmax
B. Cmax
C. Area under Curve
D. Minimum Effective Concentration

Answer: D

134. The drug concentration between Minimum Effective Concentration and Maximum Safe Concentration is called
   A. Therapeutic range
   B. Area under the curve
   C. Peak response
   D. Pharmacological response
   Answer: A

135. Tmax indicates:
   A. drug absorption rate
   B. drug elimination rate
   C. drug distribution rate
   D. drug metabolism rate
   Answer: A

136. What Will be the approximate Tmax of a drug exhibiting Ka of 2 hr-1 and K of 0.2 hr-1?
   A. 1.2 hr
   B. 2.4 hr
   C. 4.8 hr
   D. 2.0 hr
   Answer: A

137. A drug solution has a half-life of 21 days. Assuming that the drug undergoes first-order kinetics, how long will it take for the potency to drop to 90% of initial potency?
   A. 3.2 days
   B. 9.6 days
   C. 16 days
   D. 6.2 days
   Answer: A

138. Drug showing zero order kinetic of elimination
    A. Are more common than those showing first-order kinetic
    B. Show a plot of drug concentration vs time (linear Plot)
    C. Decrease in concentration exponentially with time
    D. Have half-life independent of dose
    Answer: B

139. Elimination after 4 half-lives in first-order kinetics is:
    A. 84%
    B. 93%
    C. 80%
    D. 4%
    Answer: B

140. Which one is the irrational statement for first-order kinetics?
    A. Half-life is a function of the concentration of reactants
    B. The reaction rate is not a function of the concentration of reactants
    C. Both a & b
    Answer: C

141. The half-life time of a drug can determine all of the following except
    A. Closing interval
    B. Therapeutic dose
    C. Elimination time
    D. Steady plasma concentration
    Answer: B

142. The area under the serum concentration-time curve of the drug represents
    A. The biological half-life of the drug
    B. Amount of drug biotransformed
    C. The amount of drug absorbed
    D. The amount of drug excreted in urine
    Answer: D

143. Under non-compartment analysis, the following formula is used for calculation:
A. MRT = AUMC / AUC
B. AUMC = MRT / AUC
C. MRT = AUC / AUMC
D. AUC = AUMC / MRT
Answer: A

144. Under compartment modeling, Wegner-Nelson-Method involves:
A. Determination of absorption rate constant (Ka) from %ARA vs. time curve
B. Determination of elimination rate constant (Ka) from % ARA vs. time curve
C. Determination of absorption rate constant (Ke) from %ARA vs. concentration curve
D. Determination of plasma half-life
Answer: A

145. IV infusion model follows:
A. Zero-order absorption and first-order elimination kinetic
B. No absorption and first-order elimination kinetic
C. No absorption and Zero order elimination kinetic
D. First-order absorption and first-order elimination kinetic
Answer: A

146. Select the formula to calculate the elimination half-life:
A. $t1/2 = 0.693 + Ke$
B. $t1/2 = 0.693 / Ke$
C. $t1/2 = 0.693 \times Ke$
D. $t1/2 = 0.693 - Ke$
Answer: B

147. The constants that represent the reversible transfer of drugs between
compartments are known as:
A. micro constants
B. macro constant
C. Infusion
D. Lag time
Answer: A

148. In the compartment model, the extravascular route of drug administration,
there are ………… phases:
A. absorption phase,
B. Distribution phase
C. elimination phase,
D. All of the statements are correct
Answer: D

149. Ka is estimated by:
A. Method of Residuals
B. Loo Riegelman method
C. A & B
D. None of the statements is correct
Answer: C

150. The central compartment consists of:
A. Highly perfused tissues
B. Slowly equilibrate tissues
C. Both a and b
D. Reproductive organs
Answer: A

151. A patient with severe liver disease is taking a medication primarily
metabolized by the liver. What is the most likely consequence?
A. Increased volume of distribution
B. Decreased clearance of the drug
C. Increased protein binding
D. Reduced absorption from the gut
Answer: B

152. Which of the following statements about drug interactions is true?
A. All medications taken together will interact.
B. Enzyme induction can lead to increased drug metabolism and decreased effect.
C. Competition for protein binding sites can increase free drug concentration and potential toxicity.
D. B & C
Answer: D

153. A patient with a genetic polymorphism for a drug-metabolizing enzyme is prescribed a medication with a narrow therapeutic window. What is the most crucial consideration for this patient?
A. Increasing the dosage to achieve the therapeutic effect
B. Monitoring drug levels more frequently due to the potential for increased or decreased effect
C. Switching to a medication with a wider therapeutic window
D. All of the statements are correct
Answer: D

154. AUC (Area Under the Curve) represents:
A. The peak concentration of a drug in the bloodstream
B. The total amount of drug eliminated from the body over time
C. The time it takes for the drug concentration to decrease by half
D. The extent of drug exposure over a dosing interval
Answer: D

155. Vd (volume of distribution) can be estimated using which of the following methods?
A. Noncompartmental analysis
B. Protein binding assays
C. Measurement of peak plasma concentration
D. In vitro studies
Answer: A

156. When designing a dosing regimen for a renally excreted drug, what factor
should be adjusted if a patient has decreased kidney function?
A. The dose
B. The dosing interval
C. Both dose and dosing interval
D. Neither dose nor dosing interval needs adjustment
Answer: C

157. CYP enzymes are responsible for the metabolism of many medications. Which
statement about CYP3A4 is true?
A. It is the most abundant CYP enzyme in the liver.
B. It has a narrow range of substrates it can metabolize.
C. Grapefruit juice can inhibit its activity, leading to increased drug levels.
D. Rifampin can induce its activity, leading to decreased drug levels.
Answer: C

158. Therapeutic drug monitoring (TDM) is most beneficial for medications with:
A. A wide therapeutic window
B. A narrow therapeutic window
C. High protein binding
D. Short half-life
Answer: B

159. Steady-state is achieved when:
A. The rate of drug administration equals the rate of elimination.
B. The peak plasma concentration is highest.
C. The drug is no longer detectable in the blood.
D. The medication is first administered.
Answer: A

160. Which computer program is commonly used to perform pharmacokinetic
simulations and optimize drug dosing regimens?
A. Micromedex
B. UpToDate
C. Lexi-Comp
D. WinNonLin
Answer: D

161. A pregnant woman is taking a medication that crosses the placenta. Which pharmacokinetic parameter is most important to consider for potential fetal effects?
A. Volume of distribution of the drug in the mother
B. Protein binding of the drug in the mother
C. Clearance of the drug in the fetus
D. Elimination half-life of the drug in the mother
Answer: C

162. A new medication is being investigated in a clinical trial. The researchers are using a population pharmacokinetics approach. What is the main advantage of this approach?
A. It allows for the study of drug interactions to be more effective.
B. It provides information on the pharmacokinetic variability within a population.
C. It is faster and less expensive than traditional pharmacokinetic studies.
D. It focuses solely on the safety profile of the medication.
Answer: B

163. A patient is receiving a continuous intravenous infusion of a drug. The plasma concentration of the drug reaches a plateau after a certain time. What is the reason for this plateau?
A. The drug has reached its volume of distribution.
B. The rate of elimination is equal to the rate of infusion.
C. The drug is undergoing saturation of its binding sites.
D. The patient has developed tolerance to the drug.
Answer: B

164. A medication with time-dependent pharmacokinetics exhibits a longer elimination half-life with increasing doses. What is the mechanism behind this phenomenon?
A. Saturation of metabolic pathways responsible for drug elimination.
B. Increased protein binding at higher drug concentrations.
C. Enhanced absorption from the gastrointestinal tract.
D. Reduced volume of distribution with higher doses.
Answer: A

165. Minimal residual disease (MRD) monitoring is used in some cancers. In this context, what does pharmacokinetics play a role in?
A. Selecting the most effective chemotherapy drugs.
B. Understanding the drug distribution within tumor cells.
C. Measuring the level of circulating tumor markers after treatment.
D. Optimizing the dosing regimen for targeted therapies.
Answer: C

166. Using IV infusion over 15 or 30 minutes indicates
A. Slower rate of infusion than the standard one
B. An inpatient procedure for hemorrhage-conjugated hypovolemia
C. A critical illness status
D. All of the statements are correct
Answer: D

167. Toxicity signs and symptoms after a determined drug dose intake may ensure:
A. A maximum drug concentration that exceeds MTC in multiple dosing
B. A Cmin that is below the MEC in a single IV route
C. MEC = MTC in all types of routes
D. C max at steady state in IV infusion is = C0
Answer: A

168. Biopharmaceutics is intensively concerned with the following:
A. Systemically distributed drug routes as they have no absorption PK process
B. Drug product design and development
C. Locally acting drugs such as oral liquids forms
D. Minimizing the extent of drug delivered from the drug product to achieve a safe therapeutic level for the patient
Answer: B

169. If you were informed that insulin could not be given orally, this may be justified as:
A. Insulin has low systemic bioavailability when given orally
B. Insulin is toxic when given orally
C. Insulin oral dose should be much enough (high) to overcome the degradation in GIT
D. Ulcerative GIT only may have a dysfunctioned mucosa, which leads to insufficient drug absorption
Answer: A

170. In IV bolus, Vd is:
A. Limited by cell membrane permeability
B. Affected by the active transport of the drug at the site of administration
C. Is the proportion between the dose and the concentration of the drug in plasma at that time immediately after being injected
D. Variable for the same drug when given to a targeted patient by a constant dose
Answer: C

171. A drug with consistent compatibility with the intravenous fluid:
A. Could be given in severe critical illness cases when the high liquid volume is needed
B. Could not be given as IV infusion due to the need for a slow rate of drug intake
C. Is usually toxic when used via IV routes
D. All of the statements are correct
Answer: A

172. Drug plasma concentration fluctuations:
A. May result in serious side effects
B. Could be represented through an inconsistent pharmacologic response
C. Inappropriate drug concentrations at steady state
D. All of the statements are correct
Answer: D

173. In flip-flop kinetics:
   A. When ka is much greater than k, the rate-limiting process is the elimination
   B. Irreversible first-order rate processes are the elimination and distribution
   C. Terminal lines slopes of both IV and oral routes are the same
   D. Ka and Ke are irrelevant
   Answer: A

174. A drug with an elimination half-life= 18 hr:
   A. It does not need a loading dose when given by IV infusion
   B. Loading dose is essential to reach a steady state rapidly when given as multiple dosing
   C. No need for a loading dose when given as multiple IM route
   D. Has a large elimination rate constant above 0.5
   Answer: B

175. Oral routes (single and multiple) mostly have:
   A. Rapid rate of infusion
   B. Slow rate of distribution
   C. Instant and rapid elimination
   D. None of the statements is correct
   Answer: D

176. Concerning the stomach as a significant organ for absorption:
   A. High emptying rate will elevate the rate of absorption relatively
   B. Damaged mucosa will minimize the efficiency of absorption
   C. Rapid blood flow will increase the absorption rate
   D. All of the statements are correct
   Answer: D

177. The parameters needed to establish a multiple IV dosing regimen are:
   A. The size of the drug dose
   B. MEC, MTC
   C. The frequency of drug administration
   D. All of the statements are correct
   Answer: D

A patient is started on a drug at an oral dose of 1000 mg every 4 hours. Assume a one-compartment linear model applies to this drug in this concentration range. The bioavailability of this dosage form and patient is 0.83, and the absorption rate is constant at 2.3 hr-1. The half-life and V for this drug in this patient (76 kg) are 13.9 hr and 0.27 L/kg, respectively. Please answer questions 178,179,180 and 181.

178. The elimination rate constant is:
    A. 0.0499/hr
    B. 0.5/hr
    C. 0.321/hr
    D. 0.128/hr
    Answer: A

179. The volume of distribution:
    A. 0.27L
    B. 76 L
    C. 20.5 L
    D. 3.75 L
    Answer: C

180. The concentration three hours after the first dose
    A. 0.27L
    B. 76 L
    C. 20.5 L
    D. 3.75 L
    Answer: C

181. The drug concentration one hour after the third dose is:
    A. 100.21 mg/L
    B. 77.42 mg/L L
    C. 80.52 mg/L
    D. 93.81 mg L
    Answer: D

182. The dosing interval design depends on the following:
A. Absorption half-life
B. Rate of elimination and elimination half-life
C. Volume of distribution
D. t max for the first dose (n=1)
Answer: B

183. In multiple IV dosing:
A. C(average at S.S) is the mean of Cmax (at S.S) and Cmin (at S.S)
B. C(average at S.S) could be calculated using C0 and Ke only
C. C(average at S.S) could not be calculated
D. C(average at S.S) is not the arithmetic mean of CmaxS.S, CminS.S because plasma drug concentration declines exponentially
Answer: D

184. Multiple oral dosing is quantitatively preferable to single oral dosing as:
A. Multiple oral dosing produces higher drug plasma concentrations
B. Multiple oral dosing results in lower drug plasma concentrations
C. Multiple oral dosing is qualitatively better than single oral dosing
D. Single oral dosing is qualitatively better than Multiple oral dosing
Answer: A

A drug has been given at an infusion rate of 125 mg/hr for 60 min. Two drug concentration values determined at 1.5 hr and 6 hr after the start of the infusion were 2.12 and 0.739 mg/L, respectively. Assuming a one-compartment model applies for this drug estimate the following (questions 185, 186, 187, and 188):

185. Elimination rate constant:
    A. 0.0693/hr
    B. 0.212/hr
    C. 0.15/hr
    D. 0.234/hr
    Answer: D

186. Elimination half-life:
    A. 3 hours
    B. 4 hours
    C. 5 hours
    D. 6 hours
    Answer: A

187. The volume of distribution:
    A. 15.6 L
    B. 23.4 L
    C. 46.8 L
    D. 52.3 L
    Answer: C

188. Total body clearance
    A. 11 L/hr
    B. 15.1 L/hr
    C. 10 L/hr
    D. 13.2 L/hr
    Answer: A

189. A patient was admitted to the hospital because of an acute episode of bronchial
asthma. Theophylline was administered to the patient as an IV loading dose of
300 mg, followed immediately by a constant rate IV infusion of 45 mg/hr. The
theophylline steady-state concentration achieved is 15 mg/L (k is 0.1 hr-1).
Calculate the volume of distribution.
A. 20 L
B. 30 L
C. 40 L
D. 50 L
Answer: B

190. The first-order elimination rate constant for penicillin G is 1.2 hr-1,
gentamicin is 0.35 hr-1, flucytosine is 0.1 hr-1, and rifampin is 0.2 hr-1.
Which of these drugs will reach steady-state faster during repeated
administration?
A. Penicillin G
B. Gentamicin
C. Flucytosine
D. Rifampin
Answer: A

191. A patient takes 200 mg quinidine sulfate tablet every 8 hours to treat cardiac
arrhythmia. His average plasma quinidine concentration at steady state was 2
mg/L. Because of the patient's uncontrolled condition, the physician asked you
to recommend a dosing regimen that will increase the average steady-state
plasma quinidine concentration in this patient to 6 mg/L. What will be your
recommendation?
A. 200 mg every 12 hours
B. 300 mg every 8 hours
C. 600 mg every 8 hours
D. 400 mg every 12 hours
Answer: C

192. During repeated administration of 40 mg ibuprofen tablet every 4 hours (F=1) for treating rheumatoid arthritis, the AUC during one dosing interval was 16 mg-hr/L. What is the average ibuprofen steady-state plasma concentration during this dosing regimen (40 mg every 4 hours)?

A. 2 mg/L

B. 4 mg/L

C. 5 mg/L

D. 1.5 mg/L

Answer: B

193. The following graph shows the elimination time course obtained after giving a 320 mg dose of a drug by either i.v. or oral routes. From the data displayed, the drug elimination clearance is:

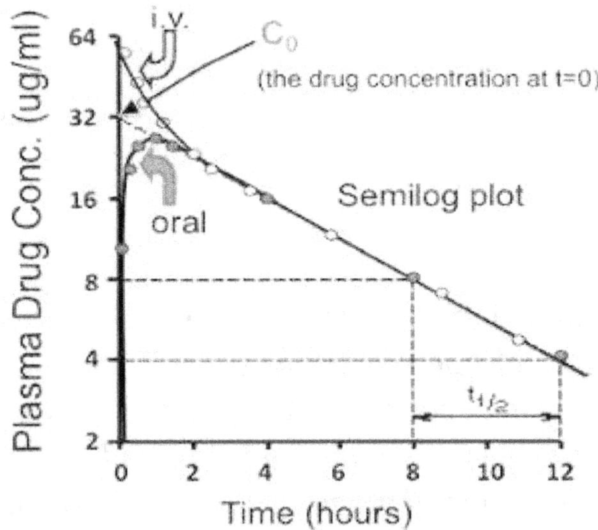

A. 0.32 L/hr

B. 1.73 L/hr

C. 10 L/hr

D. 17.3 L/hr

Answer: B

194. A 70 kg man with severe burns arrives in the Emergency Department and
requires IV Morphine to treat his pain. The Vd for morphine is 200 L. What
IV Loading dose do you need to give to rapidly achieve a therapeutic level of
60 ng/ml and relieve his pain?
A. 3 mg
B. 30 mg
C. 1.2 mg
D. 12 mg
Answer: D

A potent drug is to be given by multiple IV bolus injections. Considering the patient's clinical condition, it is decided that the Cpmax and Cpmin drug concentrations should be maintained close to but below 4 and 2 mg/L, respectively. Assume a one-compartment linear model applies to this drug in this concentration range. The Clearance and V for this drug in this patient are 9 L/hr and 61.7 L, respectively. Calculate the dosing interval that will exactly achieve this concentration requirement. Please answer questions 195, 196, 197 and 198.

195. For the previous question, the elimination rate constant is:
    A. 3.85/hr
    B. 4.75/hr
    C. 0.146/hr
    D. 0.048/hr
    Answer: C

196. The half-life for the drug in the previous question equals:
    A. 4.75 hour
    B. 3 hours
    C. 4 hours
    D. 3.5 hours
    Answer: A

197. After how many dosing intervals this drug will reach 99% of the steady-state concentration?
    A. 4.3 hour
    B. 5 hours
    C. 6.6 hour
    D. 3.3 hour
    Answer: C

198. How long will it take this drug to reach 95% of the steady state?
    A. 16.68 hour
    B. 23.75 hour
    C. 31.35 hour
    D. 20.52 hour
    Answer: D

199. The fraction (f):

A. Determines the remaining drug in the body after a specific dosing interval

B. Irrelevant to ke

C. Related to Vd

D. All of the statements are correct

Answer: A

200. Accumulation index of multiple dosing:

A. Needs to be calculated using concentrations at steady state and after the second dose

B. If the index was greater than 1, then there is an accumulation

C. Accumulation index is the same before and after the steady state

D. Could be calculated using the dose and dosing interval

Answer: B